T0196500

HOW TO BREATHE

EDWARD THOMAS HALLERAN III

authorHOUSE®

AuthorHouse™
1663 Liberty Drive
Bloomington, IN 47403
www.authorhouse.com
Phone: 1 (800) 839-8640

Published by AuthorHouse 12/18/2015

ISBN: 978-1-5049-6981-9 (sc)
ISBN: 978-1-5049-6980-2 (e)

Print information available on the last page.

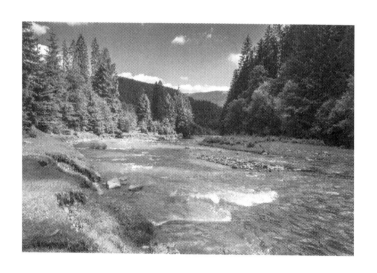

A Day in the Life

"Two Guys from Copiague"

Boats chattered nervously on tie lines, as bows bobbing in place, chewed the wooden docks. A South East wind was raising a big swell, in the Great South Bay. Two masters of the Bay arrived at their restless boat sometime after Sunrise. Let's go.

The 22 foot, decked over wooden Garvey, headed out into the wind. Most times the Bay, quiet in the morning, picked up energy throughout the Day, and laid down by Sunset; not today. This morning the Bay was an extension of the Ocean, rolling white-caps diagonally Southeast to Northwest. The little Garvey motored on, East-northeast from Babylon toward West Islip, slowing just west of Captree Bridge.

I threw anchor just South of the main Span. Immediately the craft wrenched out on the anchor line, as Cousin Tommy cut the Evinrude out-board. We were tongers. Sixteen foot pine wooden handles, tapered on one end, fit into metal baskets that bit into the Bay bottom with sharpened two and one half inch teeth. The handles, bolted above the baskets, acted like fence post diggers.

Cousin Tom had one side of the boat, I the other, we worked the edges of the deck, from bow to stern, scratching the bottom feeling for clams. Work the handles near the top, and depending on depth of water, sometimes the very top, dig and lift, dig and lift, until the basket swept under the clams and neatly closed. A shake of the basket told of clams.

On this morning the huge rolling waves smashed the bow of the embattled boat, spraying gray salt water over the shelter cabin. We were on clams thick, and continued to load the deck from bow across beam, and sides of the cabin at the stern. Skies turned ozone purplish black, gulls catching slits of sun-light above, lit the sky like white diamonds. All the other boats left the Bay, as we kept on pounding the clams.

By late morning as skies opened up, flood drains above the Bridge spewed torrents of water. As the bay turned wild, Cousin Tommy and I continued to bury the Garvey with impressive stacks of clams and coral. Suddenly, this monstrous emerald brown rogue wave breached the barrier islands into the Bay, and was rolling right at us! Without a word, Tommy lifted his tongs to mid-point on the handles, balance tipped them onto the deck; I did the same and grabbed the stretched anchor line. Tom, in big seas, nimbly tight-roped the enormous stacks, reached and fired up the outboard, gunning the boat forward. Moving past the anchor, we managed to pull it out backwards, just in time to be rising vertically, on the face of God.

*Days in our lives are complex and simple. Use the technique to breathe, and be in the moment. Cutting lawn, and stacking wood in the back-yard, I will suddenly 'hear the River'. It's been there all along.

Preface

Food. All around the World, diets are studied, relating to food, nutrition, and good health. Celebrated around the World, food is both essential to Human Life, and good Health. Without food, one may live for weeks.

Water. Gas, liquid, ice, fresh and salt, water comes in many forms, none better than cool liquid on a hot Summer day. Essential to Human life, without water one may live for days.

Oxygen. The chemistry of air we breathe, and proves, "If it is'nt impossible, it happens". Arguably, the most essential external and internal healing component experienced in Human-kind life. Without it, one may live for minutes.

The most important part of what is written here, is getting air into and out of the body. But first, one must be able to focus on the act of breathing. Sounds simple, so try this little exercise. Close your eyes, concentrate, and count back. Ten, nine, eight, seven, to zero. No other thought except the number. If any other thought interferes with the count, start over. This may take some practice, and there are many ways to clear the mind, and focus, the point being, to be single minded on the act of breathing.

Technique: We begin. Counting silently, breathe in, one thousand one, through the nose, expanding the abdomen, as if filling with air. Breathe out, one thousand one, one thousand two, through the mouth, flattening the abdomen, expelling all of the air. In front of a mirror, the air moves in through the nose, the abdomen expands, the air moves out through the mouth, the abdomen flattens. There really is no other movement. Count in thousands for rhythm. Always in a one to two ratio. In one, out two, in two, out four, in four, out eight, etc. At times hold for one count, again, for rhythm. In one thousand one, hold one thousand one, out one thousand one, one thousand two, etc. In one thousand one, one thousand two, hold one thousand one, out one thousand one, one thousand two, one thousand three, one thousand four. No particular sequence, but always in a one to two ratio, and focus on the act to optimize.

Now some poetic license.

"Spring Dream"

"Birds and budding flowers show the way, perhaps the classic robin. Warmer wind, softens Earth. Life stirs, awakens. Primal pain is felt today".

"A Great warm Friend awaits, looms vital. God breathes supple Summer wind. Earth is warmed 'till night is cool again".

"Time meets light, a curious friend. Wisdom found in the blend. Thunderous, rainbow, leaf laden wind. A dream or time machine"?

"Now the icy finger points, grimly reaching out. Store me up brittle Father, I await the slap of Life".

Discussion

So, contained in the air are the molecules that heal both internally and externally. Change the chemistry, add more oxygen. Vibrate it. Salt-air, near the Ocean. Respiratory dis-ease is caused, by the lack of it. More air is Good.

*One for the Planet: "If litter were dollar bills, there would'nt be any, so pick it up".

*One for Capitalism: "Not having money; the root of all evil.

*One for Fun: "When you don't know where you are going in a hurry, you get lost faster".

*One for Wisdom: "If a man or woman expects more from anyone, other than that they are here, they expect too much".

Summary

I like to sit, facing the Ocean. Relax. The Ocean breeze, and salt-air. Where the water meets the sand, sea foam. I close my eyes and see, Red Snapper, lobster, and blue crab. Yellow and blue-fin tuna, the Great White, and Orca. The Graceful Blue Whale. The Horizon. Many disciplines, help us to focus. The sole focus is to Breathe.

Expand, and Contract. Count silently. In, one thousand one, through the nose, the belly expands, as if filling with the air. Out, one thousand one, one thousand two, through the mouth, the belly flattens, expelling all of the air. In one, out two. In two, out four. In one thousand one, one thousand two, one thousand three; Out one thousand one, one thousand two, one thousand three, one thousand four, one thousand five, one thousand six. Expand and contract. At times, hold for one count for rhythm. With focus, and correctly done, arrive in the Moment, the only time anything in the History of Mankind, has ever happened!!!

Mathematically speaking, the chemistry of air, is nearly impossible. In other words, enjoy the miracle of both external and internal healing. At rest meditate. At work energize. Working out, recover. When you fatigue, rejuvenate. The children find "How to Breathe", better than candy. First grade, in every school, in every Country, on every Continent, would be better for it.

Finally: Six thousand, nine hundred languages, known. Humankind breathes, all in One. Seven billion, and no-one left out. One Source, for All.

"To breathe, or not to breathe", is to Be or Not to Be. So, "I Breathe, therefore, I Am".

Take Care, and be Care-full;

With Love, Papa Edge.

The core value of "How to Breathe", is the act of focusing on getting air into, and out of the body. While not as flashy as jumping from an airplane, it will just as surely get you into the Moment. Nothing happens yesterday, nor does it happen tomorrow. What-ever it is, it all happens now, in the Present Moment. There really can be no more an exciting time, and the technique, and focus on this simple act, will get you 'there'. While Gourmet restaurants, take the act of eating life sustaining food to an art form, something is amiss. Awesome polar caps, and Oceans, rivers, and the cycle of life sustaining water, still leaves something to be desired. It is in the air, and how we process that, allowing us to fully appreciate, everything else.

Sometimes when we consider, looking inside an invisible atom, or speck of energy, and find smaller things, and then the invisible portion of that being the life force, and then out, at 186,000 thousand miles per second, the speed of light, and 13.7 billion years, we find ourselves in DEEP Space. Consider that light would circle Earth, 7.5 times in one second, and some of the stars we gaze up at night are bigger than our Sun, light years away, and more plentiful than grains of sand on the beach. Let us zoom back in, and step into our own shoes. We are all part of something big, and may participate in the un-folding of a UNIVERSE!!!!!

All that from the simple act of "How to Breathe"? Just observing from the only time, 'it', is all happening. "A day in the Life", is meant to be a day in any one of our lives. All of the rest of the writing is to support the premise, and medical doctors concur, "How we feel, effects, how we Breathe". Therefore, how we breathe, effects, how we feel. It is really not at all, too selfish. To focus, or meditate, on the simple act of getting more air into, and out of our bodies, is part of the larger living Planet.

So heal both internally and externally, and enjoy the Eternal Moment.

EDGE.

About the Author

Grew up on the South Shore of Long Island, New York. Irish and Italian, so loves beer and pasta. Drove one and a half million miles around the Country-side, and thinks America is the Greatest Place on Earth. Favorite animal is the Thoroughbred Race-Horse. Thinks life may exist some-where else in the Universe, but still believes Women to be God's greatest Creation.

Printed in the United States
By Bookmasters